KETO MINDSET

How to lose weight in 30 days on a Ketogenic diet. Simple steps to Keto success, giving you the best advice and motivation needed from a coach allowing you to achieve long-term results

By Gabriel Walker

Table of Contents

Introduction

When I was young, I was that person who ate like an elephant but never picked up weight. That was until I got into my early 20s. As a female, the older you get, the more difficult it is to let go of those few extra pounds. I struggled!

I looked up every diet I could and followed it. I remember trying crazy diets like the Weet-Bix diet and the coffee and no food diet. I even tried water fasting and so many other options, all to no avail. I would stand on the scale and cry every time.

After successfully completing a diet, I quickly ended up picking all that weight right back up again. One day, as I was browsing the Internet, I came across the keto diet. It was something that I didn't really understand at first. It looked like stuff I would love to eat and not the type of food that would send me running for the hills.

After no longer trusting anything I read on the Internet, I was ready to give up and throw in the towel for good. Not long after that my SMS tone went off, and there was a high school reunion coming up that following weekend. I was very anxious to see everyone again. I met up with one of a good friend from high school that very same day, wondering if she would judge the way I looked since I used to be known as the skinny one. When I laid my eyes on her, my jaw dropped! Never in my life would I have thought that my friend whom I haven't seen in a few months was standing right in front of me. She looked amazing! She had lost so much weight, and it was scary!

During our conversation, she informed me about the keto diet and that she was one of the many success stories out there. Then she handed me a handful of sites to visit. I read everything and broke it down for you as much as I could.

I became a keto diet success story myself, and if I can do it, then so can you. But before we even get there, you need to understand why I decided to write this book for you, the readers. I want you to be able to fully understand how your body works and why it is so essential to maintain a healthy lifestyle.

In this book, I am also going to give you my 30-day keto diet plan so that you can start somewhere too. When you do decide to dedicate yourself to this diet, keep in mind it's going to be very hard at first. But I am here to help you along the way. Rome was not built in a day, so be patient with yourself.

I have also included a section on how to increase your metabolism and a few weight loss tips I picked up along the way. If you follow my guide, you are guaranteed to have a long and healthy life with long term results. This is not one of those quick fix me up diets; after a while, it becomes a part of your lifestyle.

Another thing to remember is that when you start any type of diet, it's crucial to also exercise if you haven't already been doing so. Also, if you have a cheat day, don't be too hard on yourself. Generally, people who accidentally or purposely cheat on a diet feel guilty about occasionally having something sweet.

Luckily with this diet, you never have to worry about cheating! Therefore, you will not overeat or do anything you are not supposed to. That is the beauty of this diet. The keto diet is one that will change your life.

I will also suggest some healthy snacks that you can have because I know how difficult it can be in the beginning stages. Eventually, you won't even need these suggestions.

Take my weight loss tips into consideration because I think they are essential to know before you start doing anything. Remember that reliable sites give out recipes too. Once your 30 days are up, you can start moving to other types of keto foods.

Before we even get started, you are probably wondering, "what is a keto diet?" A keto diet is a plan of meals that are very low in carbohydrates. You lower your carbohydrate intake to under 100 grams a day.

This makes it very easy to abolish junk food and all types of heavy processed products. It's important you understand that this is not just a temporary diet; this leads to a lifestyle change.

This is ideal for people with diabetes, people who are overweight or obese, people with many other health reasons, and more! In order for me to prove to you that this diet indeed works, I am going to have to jump into some biology.

Your body's energy

We, as human beings, need the energy to keep us alive. Food breaks down in our bodies and is turned into useable energy. This energy makes us feel awake during the day. The human body has a few places where it gets its energy sources from; some are stored in your body's fats and some in your ketones.

Your body also takes glucose from the liver and all your carbohydrates from the food you eat. Now you may be wondering what will happen if we were to take the carbohydrates away because they are the primary source of energy in your body.

Let me explain this in the simplest way I can.

After you eat your carbs and they enter your bloodstream, they are broken down into glucose. Then, insulin steps in to try and get rid of all the extra glucose from your blood. It takes your glucose and transforms it into glycogen, which is stored primarily in your body's muscles.

This becomes a problem when you don't exercise because the glycogen gets stored in your muscles. When all your muscles are full, and your liver is full, then it sends out a signal to stop the production of insulin.

The glycogen has nowhere to go at this point, so more insulin is released, and eventually, this leads to insulin resistance. When your body reaches this point, the liver sends any left-over glucose to be stored as body fat (Lis, 2019).

This is when you start to gain weight and can develop type 2 diabetes and many other metabolic issues.

Keto snacks

One dill pickle	One slice of bacon	One beef stick	Two stalks of celery
One tablespoon of guacamole	Fifteen pecan nuts	One keto bar	A handful of cherry tomatoes
One hard-boiled egg	One mini round of Babybel cheese	Eight brazil nuts	One piece of string cheese

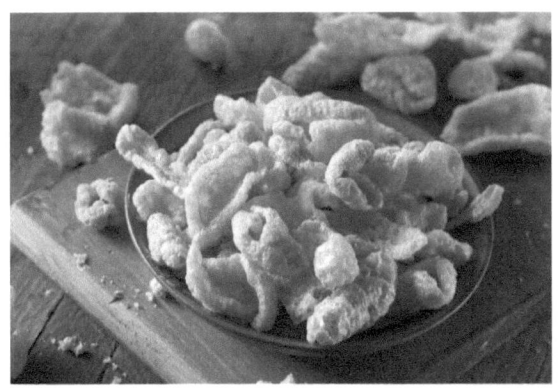

These are just some of many snacks. These are my go to's because they are my favourites. You can also find different types of snacks; you just have to look them up. Preferably only read the sites that are approved by dieticians. Here are some more snacks that you need to eat in moderation. It all depends on the diet you have.

Below I have compiled a list of grab-to-go snacks. These don't need any preparation, and you can just grab them from your refrigerator when you are hungry.

Olives	Sugar-free jelly
Sugar-free ice cream	Kale chips
Iced coffee	Pork rinds
Sardines	Seaweed snacks
Avocado	Stevia sweetened dark chocolate
Pepperoni slices	Beef jerky
Laughing cow cheese	Macadamia nuts

Below I have compiled a list of the snacks you can make at home. You can find the recipes for them on Google. These do require a bit of preparation, but it is worth it in the long run.

Steak tips	Keto fries
Pizza	Bone broth
Fat bombs	Flaxseed crackers
Keto pate	Keto crisps
Calzones	Salad

Like I mentioned before, these are just some of many snacks. There are many types of snacks, but these are the most popular ones. As you can see, there are many snacks that you fall back on if you get hungry while on this diet.

Remember, a keto diet is a low carbohydrate diet with high-fat content. With this diet, you can reverse type 2 diabetes and treat epilepsy (Lis, 2019), and if that's not why you are here, that's okay too.

This diet is guaranteed weight loss for anyone. The above mentioned are just a bonus!

Chapter 1- Keto diet weight loss tips

Below is a list of weight loss tips, written by Eenfeldt (2019), that are important to follow before, during, and after the diet. These tips helped me better understand a few things when it came to losing weight. I am sure it will do the same for you.

These tips are here to motivate you and encourage you to do the best that you can. Just a friendly warning, you might not see much of a difference in your weight in the first two weeks. This is completely normal. Don't give up, because like I said, these things take time.

1.   Be persistent

I am going to be super blunt in saying forget about all of those "quick fixes." There is no magic cure to losing weight. It comes with hard work and dedication. You can't simply take a magic pill that will drop those extra pounds overnight. There is absolutely no such thing. It's rubbish and dangerous. So, stay away from those.

Whatever you do, don't starve yourself and think that it is a long-term solution. Starving yourself is dangerous and can lead to bulimia. Don't even attempt to starve yourself just a little bit. This is a horrible way to think you will lose weight successfully.

As soon as you put food in your mouth, your body is going to store that food away because your body does not know when it will get food again. This causes weight gain, and it is simply a bad thing to do to yourself and your body.

You need to understand that your weight did not magically appear on your body overnight. This weight you have on your body has been growing there for many years. It's nothing to be ashamed of, you are reading this for help, and I am going to give it to you. Just be patient with your body; results take time.

Let's get one thing straight, if you want to keep your weight off permanently, you need to change your habits and your lifestyle forever. It's not something you do for a short time and expect it to work. Once you change your lifestyle, everything else will fall into place.

Like I mentioned before, if you don't see a change in the first two weeks, please don't panic. We are all different, and sometimes it takes our bodies longer to adapt to the change. Other people are lucky enough that they start losing weight within the first week.

Work towards losing 1-3kg in the first week. As I said, everyone is different, but work towards that. After that you should be losing half a kilogram a week, all depending on how much excess weight you still have on your body.

You will be happy to know that every kilogram you lose in weight, you lose a centimetre around your bust.

2. Avoid fruit

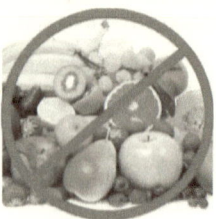

Unfortunately, all fruit has sugar that shuts down your fat burning cells in your body. So, it would be best to avoid fruit altogether. When you are eating fruit regularly, it increases your desire to eat, therefore causing your weight loss to slow down rapidly.

If you haven't already guessed it, fruit itself contains a concerning amount of sugar, and we want to stay away from that if we're going to lose weight. Did you know that five servings of fruit contain as much sugar as a 500ml soft drink? That means that sugar is about 50% glucose and 50% fructose.

3. Eat only when hungry

If you eat when you are hungry, you will be able to limit the need for unnecessary snacking. If you are not hungry during lunchtime, then don't eat lunch. You are more than welcome to skip meals. Try your best not to overeat. This is very easy to do with peanuts.

4. Review your medicine

The very first thing you need to do when you start your weight loss journey is to check your blood pressure, cholesterol levels, and your sugar to make sure that you are in good health. Many medications can contribute to your struggle of losing weight.

Insulin-releasing tablets	Some contraception medication
Cortisone	Antibiotics

Antipsychotic drugs	Epilepsy drugs
Some anti-depressants	Allergy medication
Insulin injections	Blood pressure drugs

5. Eat less dairy and nuts

Dairy products slow down weight loss if consumed in large quantities. Nuts, especially salty ones, are very easy to keep eating without realising how much you are consuming. This could be dangerous, as too much salt is not healthy for you either.

6. Supplement vitamins and minerals

It is nearly impossible to get all the vitamins and minerals we need every single day from just consuming food. Go out and get yourself a high-quality multivitamin that you can take every day. Did you know that it is quite difficult to get vitamin D? The funny thing is that vitamin D is the key to weight loss.

So, look up the right amount of vitamin D that you need to take every single day and buy some in pill form. It should be widely available wherever you are around the world.

7. Support during your journey

If you are anything like me, you are going to need all the help you can get from friends and family. Have a family meeting and invite your friends over as well. Tell them what you plan to do and how you are planning to do it.

You never know, your family might decide to join you. The more, the merrier! Once they have all been informed, ask your family and friends for support. Let them know that they are now your pillars. Ask them to encourage you.

8. Exercise

Your body needs at least one hour of aerobic exercise if you are just starting out. But remember to take it slow and don't overdo it. You still want to be able to walk the next day. If you can, get yourself a smartwatch that tracks the number of steps you take each day.

The average steps for a woman daily is around 10,000 steps. If you are not new to the concept of exercise and you have been consistently doing it, look into joining a dance class or start playing a new sport like tennis.

Remember that exercise is essential every single day!

9.   Check your hormones

If you struggle with losing weight and shedding off those few extra pounds, you should consider getting your thyroid checked. Stress levels, as well as your sex hormones, need to be checked as well. You might not be losing anything due to one of these three problems.

Believe it or not, your hormones play a huge role when it comes to losing weight. If anything is slightly off, it will break your body's equilibrium, and it will not function the way it should. That is why it is imperative to make sure you get these checked as often as possible.

Don't put this off for long; make sure you get regular checkups. Many people don't understand how important these checkups actually are. They could make the world's difference.

10.   Avoid your weekend beer

I personally don't like beer, but many people do. It's better you avoid that weekend beer. That doesn't mean don't drink anything. If you are a man, indulge yourself in some old whiskey. Ladies, stay away from that wine too, have some vodka instead.

Like fruit, beer contains rapidly digested carbs that shut down the fat burning cells in your body. So, you should stay away from the beer altogether. Alcohol, in general, needs to be taken in moderation.

11.   Choose a low carb diet

Studies have shown that when you are on a low carb diet, you burn calories even while you are resting or sleeping. How amazing is that? You can burn up to three hundred calories doing nothing but closing your eyes. You don't even need to move!

Being on a low carb diet means that you need to avoid foods that contain starch and sugar, which includes potatoes, bread, and pasta. The main advantage of a low carb diet is that it makes you full for longer, therefore causing you to eat less. A low carb diet will make you want to eat less in general.

It is also scientifically proven that a low carb diet is the healthiest and most effective way to lose weight. That's why it is best to adopt a low carb diet over any other diet.

12.   Determine if you are really hungry

In today's busy world, even with things changing around us every second, a person can still get bored. Typically, when you are bored and have nothing to do, you start to feel hungry. It's a common feeling for people, especially young adults. You need to make sure that you are not just eating because you have nothing better to do.

Stress is a horrible thing to have. There is absolutely no way to avoid it. There is not a single person on this planet who is not stressed out. You need to see that you are not eating due to stress. Stress eating is like comfort to some people. Try and avoid stress eating at all costs.

Once you have ruled out that you are not doing any of the above, you can then confirm that you are actually hungry and that your body needs food. This tip goes hand in hand with the tip #3. This is helpful to know so that you can decipher if you are really hungry or not.

13.   Stress less

Try yoga or meditation to help ease your restless mind. Meditation doesn't have to take up so much of your time either, 3 to 5 minutes a day to yourself will do you good. Another effective way to de-stress is to pick up a book and read.

Stress releases a horrible hormone called cortisol. This hormone makes you incredibly hungry and causes a substantial change in a person's appetite. This hunger, in the long run, will cause weight gain instead of weight loss.

A respectable amount of relaxation is vital when it comes to staying away from stress. If you feel well rested, you tend to be less stressed out. This, in the long run, will help you avoid stress.

14.   Sleep correctly

I am not talking about the way you sleep or the position you sleep in at night. I am talking about the amount of sleep and rest that you get out of it. Remember that you need to get at least fifteen minutes of sunlight a day, not just to get your daily dose of the sun, but it actually contributes to your rest.

If you are a coffee lover, such as myself, I have some bad news for you. Avoid coffee or any sort of caffeine after 1 in the afternoon because caffeine takes forever to leave your system. Also, it would be a great idea to set a bedtime so that you can set a regular routine for yourself.

Rest is vital to losing weight. Once you are in routine, stick to it. This tip goes hand in hand with our previous tip. The point is to avoid stress and get your body relaxed to prevent that stress hormone from being released.

Do not exercise right before you go to bed, as this will keep your body awake, and you will miss out on your beauty sleep. If you have to exercise in the evening, make sure you do so at least four hours before you need to go to sleep.

15. Intermittent fasting

Before we get started with this, I must warn you. Don't do this if you are under the age of 18.

Young people should definitely not be doing this as it is not good for their health.

Don't take part in intermittent fasting if you are on any form of medication as this could cause complications for your health. Do not attempt this if you have been diagnosed with chronic stress; this could cause you to faint or pass out.

Lastly, do not attempt this if you suffer from sleep deprivation; this could lead to severe complications. If none of the above applies to you, you can keep reading. You can keep up with intermittent fasting for as long as you'd like to, so long as you are in good health.

You can do this once a week or every day for a month; the choice is all yours. So, let me break this down for you as much as I can so it's not complicated to understand. The easiest way to do this is to not eat for 16 hours of the day. This includes the hours that you are sleeping. Many people fast from 8pm to 12pm. This means that a person's first meal of the day will be at lunch. You get the idea.

16. Track your progress

I think that everyone should already know that you should take your measurements before you start on your weight loss journey. After you start your journey, you should only take measurements once a month.

The best time to take your measurements is the very first thing in the morning to get the most accurate results. Your body mass index is the best way to track your weight loss. You don't want to be underweight for your height and age.

The first thing to do is to step on the scale and write down your weight on a piece of paper or in a notebook. After that, grab a measuring tape (the ones they use for sewing) and place it slightly above your belly button. Take a deep breath in and out. Don't try and suck in that tummy of yours! I am watching you!

Make sure the tape fits snug and is not compressing your skin because then you are only cheating yourself. Remember not to feel discouraged; these things take time. Take your measurement in centimetres and write it down.

Remember that for every kilogram you lose, you will lose a centimetre around your bust too!

17. Weight loss pills

If you have been dieting and it has not been working, only resort to pills as a last resort. Remember, I mentioned that there is no such thing as a magic pill that will make your weight suddenly drop.

It will never make you thin overnight. I'm not saying that these tablets don't work, they do, but only temporarily. Once you stop taking these tablets, all the weight you lost comes back just as quick as you lost it. Most of these weight loss pills are utter rubbish.

The ingredients can cause nasty side effects as well, so take all of this into consideration before deciding to take the first pill you see. You need to do proper and thorough research to make sure what you swallow isn't going to kill you.

18.   Avoid artificial sweeteners

Artificial sweeteners are probably one of the most dangerous products that you can use when it comes to losing weight. They increase a person's appetite immensely and create intense cravings for sweet food. This can also create a bad addiction to sugar, so do your best to steer clear of them.

When I say artificial sweeteners, this includes all and any types of sodas. Diet sodas included, believe it or not. Diet sodas create insulin in your body. This could be very bad for any person; it could lead you to developing type 2 diabetes.

Consumption of artificial sweeteners can be deadly for people with type 1 diabetes. It's best to stay away from any type of sweeteners, artificial or not. It's all dangerous and harmful to your body.

The importance of maintaining a healthy lifestyle

Many people don't consider their lifestyle when they plan to lose weight. In fact, your lifestyle plays a vital role. We as human beings have different views on what a healthy lifestyle is; in our case, it is reaching our optimal physical as well as mental being.

In this day, humans have evolved into leading a lifestyle with very unhealthy habits. Let's be honest with one another, we can live better lifestyles without these habits. These bad habits include smoking cigarettes,drugs, as well as drinking teamed up with very poor and inactive physical activity. This has led us humans to adopt lousy quality diets as well.

To lose weight, you need regular physical activity. So be sure to make yourself a schedule and stick to it. Sleep and rest also play a significant role when it comes to losing those few extra pounds and leading a healthy lifestyle.

Leading a healthy lifestyle is vital for many reasons, including disease prevention. If you do not exercise daily, it leads to sickness and chronic illnesses. Being sick leads you to gain weight due to antibiotics and not getting enough physical exercise.

Leading a healthy lifestyle is important because if you don't watch what you put in your mouth, it can lead you to eat poorly and will cause you to have a chronic poor diet; and if you have a poor diet, you are very likely to pick up various diseases like type 2 diabetes.

If you develop type 2 diabetes, there is a considerable chance that you will gain a lot of weight because insulin releasing medications cause weight gain. You will then also be at risk for heart problems in the near future.

Maintaining a healthy lifestyle is vital to reducing stress and adding on a few more valuable years to your life. This leads me to tell you that if you maintain a healthy lifestyle, you can improve your overall health which includes your mental health.

Important exercises to help you lose weight

Now that we have established that exercising is essential, I would like to share a few weight loss exercises with you. But before I do that, you should know that weight loss exercises are also known as cardiovascular exercises.

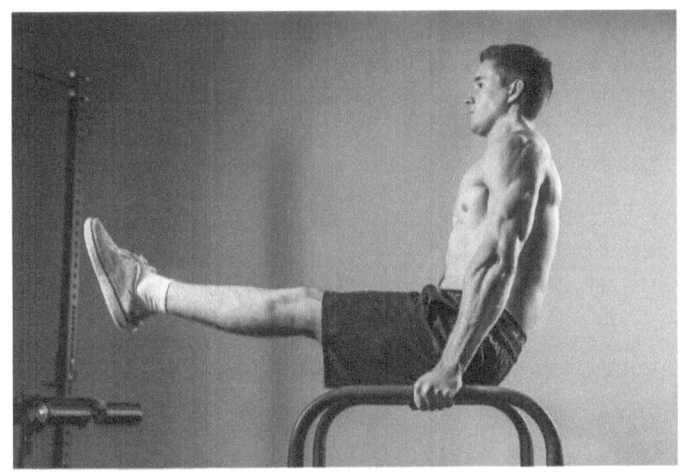

The first thing we look at when we want to start training is aerobic exercises. The point of this is to increase your heart rate. This doesn't necessarily mean that you have to run a marathon; it can be walking and swimming too.

Do note that you need to consult your doctor or a personal trainer before attempting exercises on your own. When you are on a low carb diet, you can't dive into extreme exercises without the approval of a professional as it can cause complications.

When you adopt a low carb diet, it puts a lot of stress on your body, so when you do decide to finally exercise, it's important that you listen to your body. You don't want to put yourself in danger just for the sake of losing weight faster.

Please for heaven's sake, make sure you eat enough! Remember, exercising burns carbohydrates first, so you have to be sure that you have enough healthy fats to keep you going.

The first few weeks of your diet are going to be intense, so you should really take it easy by completing low-intensity exercises. This diet works, but I never said it was going to be easy, because if I did, I would be lying to you.

It is challenging to walk past that bakery aisle with all the freshly baked doughnuts and cakes, and it is probably going to drive you insane. But remember why you are doing this. Remember that going on a diet should be for yourself and not anyone else.

Let's take a look at some workouts you can do in a pool. A cardio workout in a pool is pretty simple. When you do decide to go swimming, make sure you follow all the rules when it comes to using a public or gym pool. Swim for five continuous minutes and take a break at the edge of the pool for thirty seconds. Then, grab a kickboard and kick continuously for five minutes. Repeat this exercise three times for a full body and cardio workout (Scott, 2019).

If swimming really isn't your thing, go out and buy a good quality jump rope. Jump for half an hour a day and you are set for a friendly and easy cardio workout. If you have access to a gym, it will probably be best to do some rowing. However, don't overdo it, just row for a little while.

If you have been exercising for a long time and you are comfortable to try more intense training, and you have approval from your doctor or trainer, you can do the following.

If you prefer to exercise at home, I am going to give you my workout plan. You can take twominute breaks as often as you need to throughout these exercises. The first exercise I usually start with is squats, and I do one hundred and fifty of them. Remember that you can take as many two-minute breaks as you need in between each exercise.

I then proceed to do one hundred lunges, with breaks in-between. Once that is finished, and I have caught my breath, I do one hundred jumping jacks, and eighty leg raises. Once I have caught my breath again, I finish off with some running.

There is an app in the Apple app store that you can download for free. It is called "The Beep Test." The point of the beep test is to reach the finish line before you hear the beep. The speed increases after each beep making the exercise more and more difficult.

Chapter 2- Allowed list of foods for Keto

Now that you have the basics covered, you are probably wondering what exactly it is that you are allowed to eat. Below I am going to share everything I know when it comes to the foods that pass the keto friendly test.

You will be amazed by how many common foods you can eat if you switch around a few of the ingredients. But before I get there, let's start off with the types of meat you are allowed to eat.

You can still have a decent restaurant breakfast anywhere you go because the keto diet is simply that amazing. Take a look below.

Bacon	Cold cuts
Lamb	Fowl
Pork	All red meat
Chicken	Turkey

That might not look like much, but it really is a lot. You will be amazed to know how much fish and seafood you can have as well. I am personally a significant fan of fish, especially squid, so I was happy to learn that I could still eat my favourite seafood. If you are allergic to fish, feel free to skip this section.

All fish	Squid
Scallops	Clams
Oysters	Muscles
Lobster	Shrimp
Crabs	Crawfish

At the beginning of chapter one, I instructed you to avoid fruit at all costs. However, this does not mean that you have to avoid fruit forever. Once you have reached your goal weight, you are more than welcome to start introducing fruit back into your diet; however, do it slowly.

I must admit, I missed avocado for the first few months; but let me tell you, when I got to eat it again, it tasted even better. Consume of these fruits with strict moderation obviously. The keto diet doesn't eliminate everything you love forever, just until you have reached a state of ketosis.

Here is a list of acceptable fruits that you can eat after you have reached your goal.

Raspberries	Strawberry
Lemon	Avocado
Lime	Apricot
Grapefruit	Blackberry

Here is one for all the cheese lovers out there. There is a wide variety of cheeses that you can eat. There are so many options for you to wrap in cold cuts and enjoy! Again, this is all to be taken in moderation. Here are the keto accepted cheeses.

Cheddar	Gouda
Provolone	Mozzarella
Neufchatel	Ricotta
Gruyere	Blue cheese
Parmesan	Fontina
Muenster	Edam
Monterey	Havarti

Next up is a list of salad dressings and fats that you are allowed to have. Most of them have a limit of two tablespoons which still goes incredibly well over a salad of your choice.

Butter	Mayonnaise
Blue cheese dressing	Olive oil
Italian dressing	Avocado oil
Caesar dressing	Coconut oil
Ranch dressing	1000 island dressing

The keto diet even supports those who've adopted a vegan lifestyle. I have compiled a list of vegan protein that you may have if you have decided to live that lifestyle.

Soybeans	Soymilk
Soy nuts	Firm tofu
Tempeh	Silken tofu

There is nothing I love more when it comes to vegetables. You have no idea how ecstatic I was when I found a list of all the veggies I can eat. It is an overwhelming amount, and that made me so happy.

Below I have compiled a list of the many veggies you can have!

Bamboo shoots	Asparagus	Artichoke hearts in water	Artichoke	Romaine lettuce	Radishes
Pumpkin	Okra	Kohlrabi	Daikon	Endive	Radicchio
Onion	Black olives	Leeks	Alfalfa sprouts	Escarole	Bell peppers
Sauerkraut	Spinach	Mushrooms	Broccoli	Arugula	Parsley
Cherry tomato	Tomato	Kale	Brussels sprouts	Bok choy	Jicama
Turnips	Collard greens	Hearts of palm	Cabbage	Celery	Iceberg Lettuce
Green onions	Chard	Eggplant	Cauliflower	Chicory greens	Fennel

Cucumber					

Did you know that with a keto diet you can use all and any spices? If you have cholesterol problems, please don't overuse your salt. It is unhealthy for you.

Moving on, I am going to give you the list that I have compiled for dairy products. This list is a bit short but still worth mentioning.

Unsweetened almond milk	Full fat sour cream	Plain full greek yogurt
Heavy whipping cream	Whole eggs	Egg whites and egg yolk

Now that we have covered all the basics, I am going to add a little extra information in for you to know about. I have also compiled a lovely list of nuts and seeds that you can consume. Unfortunately, the same rule applies as it does to fruit; you should only eat them if you've reached ketosis.

Once you have reached your goal weight, you are more than welcome to start introducing nuts and seeds back into your diet; do so slowly. Here is a list of acceptable nuts and seeds that you can use after you have reached your goal weight.

Peanut butter	Almond butter
Pumpkin seeds	Sunflower seeds
Walnuts	Pistachio nuts
Almonds	Pine nuts
Peanuts	Pecans
Hazelnut	Macadamia nuts

Now that all of our solids have been listed, it's time to move on to liquids. We are going to start off with alcoholic beverages that don't contain carbohydrates. Yes, that's right. Alcohol is keto approved.

Tequila	Gin
Whiskey	Vodka
Rum	Martini

As I mentioned before, beer is a huge no-no; it is like eating loaves of bread one after another. Stick to the list of alcoholic beverages above, and you can still have fun while celebrating special occasions. Next, we have a list of acceptable standard drinks.

Water	Herbal tea
Unsweetened tea	Unsweetened coffee
No calorie flavored seltzers	Sugar-free sparkling water
Diet soda (watch for sweeteners)	Club soda

Now that we have completed the section on foods and drinks that we are allowed to have, the next section is about the foods that we have to stay away from in order to lose weight and reach our goals.

Banned list of foods for Keto

Now, you are probably going to hate what you see here, and sadly the truth hurts, so get ready to have the biggest shock of your life when you finally see everything we are not allowed to eat. Hold on to your seats ladies and gentlemen, this is going to be a rough ride.

Considering we ended on drinks in the previous section, I thought it would be best to start this section off with the drinks we are not allowed to have. This includes alcoholic and nonalcoholic beverages. Here we go.

Wine coolers	Alcopops
Sweetened or flavoured coffee	Sweet cocktails

Sweetened or flavoured tea	Energy drinks
All sweetened drinks	Frozen coffee beverages
Soda	Malt
Juice	Root beer floats
Frappuccino Coffee drinks	Milkshakes

I was so surprised to see that there were so many things that we can't eat when it comes to grains and starches that you normally have with a regular carbohydrate diet. I am going to divide this list into two parts. Let's first have a look at part one.

All whole grains	Any fried food	Whole wheat flour
Oatmeal	French Toast	Rice flour
Cream of wheat	Pasta	Corn flour
Pancakes	Bread	White flour
Waffles	Bagels	Corn starch
Pizza	English muffins	Pasta
Porridge	Croissants	White rice
Barley	Tortilla	Cold breakfast cereals

You will see that the list above contains a lot of baking ingredients and quite a few starches. It is vital that you don't eat any of these as they are not suitable for you and will bring you out of ketosis. Let's now have a look at part two.

Crackers	Muesli
Amaranth	Rye

Millet	Spelt
Quinoa	Bulgur

I put these items in part two because these food items are common misconceptions, in the sense that they are easily mistaken for what some people would call "healthy." They obviously are not. Since we're on the topic of unhealthy foods, I think it's time to move on to the list of fruits you should never eat while on a keto diet.

Dried fruit	Oranges
Kiwifruit	Applesauce
Pears	Dates
Pomegranates	Pears
Pineapple	Plums
Cherries	Figs
Grapes	Banana
Mango	Tangerines

All of these fruits have a high amount of sugar in them, and some even contain starch. It is best to avoid them as much as possible if you want to keep the excess weight off. I have also compiled a list of fruits that contain medium levels of sugar as well as starch-filled fruits.

Apricots	Guava
Honeydew melons	Grapefruit
Apples	Peaches
Nectarines	Papaya
Watermelons	Cantaloupes

Blueberries	

I also compiled a list of vegetables you should not consume. Take a look below.

Lentils	Pinto beans
Lima beans	Baked beans
Black beans	Chickpeas
Kidney beans	Navy beans

If you are not lactose intolerant, you are probably wondering which dairy products we should not consume. You will find that your days for comfort food are over. Here is a hint, no more ice cream!

Ice cream	Yogurt with fruit pieces and sugar
Flavoured dairy	Cottage cheese
Whole and skim milk	Pudding
Soymilk (if you are not a vegan)	Margarine

Now that we are on the topic of comfort foods, there are a few sweets and packaged snacks that we should stay away from. There are also a few processed foods included in there. Remember that all other candy not listed below is also included, as well as all other boxed snacks.

Cupcakes	Twinkies
Cotton candy	Granola bars
Hard candy	Pop-tarts
Chocolate bars	Popcorn

Flavoured nuts	Potato crisps
Pretzels	Tortilla crisps
Rice cakes	Raisins
Breakfast bars	Cheese and cracker snacks

I am going to end this section off with the obvious: you should avoid eating any sugar even if you are not on a diet. This includes all and any types of sugars, honey included, as well as baked goods like cookies and cakes.

Ten common keto mistakes

There are ten common errors that can occur when it comes to losing weight and sticking to a low carb diet.

Overeating protein	Being afraid of fat
Not eating enough	Not exercising
Not eating enough veggies	Being afraid to eat out
Not giving the body enough time to adjust	Listen to friendly advice
Allowing boredom to sabotage your efforts	Not replenishing sodium

Please take the following into consideration. The keto diet allows you to eat eggs; however, that does not mean five or six eggs a day. This will compromise your diet for too much protein. We want to keep with the recommended daily protein.

In order for you to exercise correctly and be healthy, you need to have natural and healthy fats. Don't be afraid of fats; they are good for you. Don't try and get rid of all fats because your body needs them in order for it to function normally.

People think that when they are on this diet plan that they are not meant to eat a lot of food.

That is a common mistake made by many people. You have to eat as much as is necessary so that you don't pass out or cause severe damage to your body. It is crucial that you eat!

Remember that lovely long list of veggies I gave you earlier? You know you don't have to eat them raw, right? Use spices and melt the right amount of recommended cheese over top of them! This is allowed. Just make sure you eat an appropriate serving of veggies.

Like I said before, Rome was not built in a day. You have to give your body time to adjust. It is a life-altering diet and to make sure you get the results you want, you're going to have to be patient and give your body all the time it needs to adjust.

This also means that you have to be mindful throughout this process; you are working hard to make a lifestyle change, so don't let your efforts be destroyed by boredom or stress. I used to eat a lot when I was stressed, and unfortunately, that was my biggest downfall. Don't allow this to happen to you too!

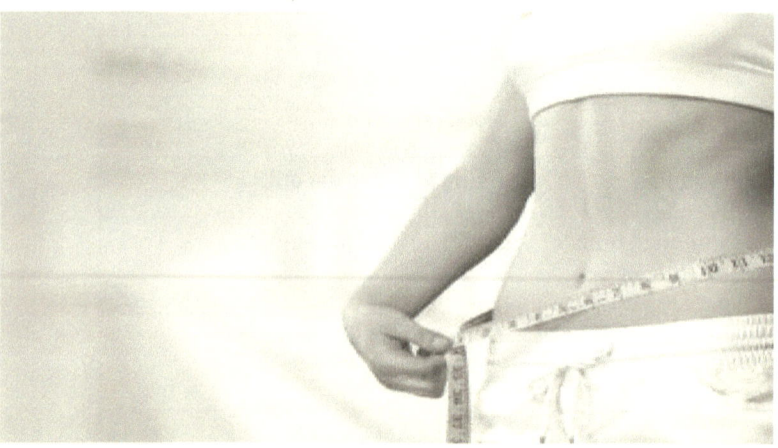

Many people are going to want to give you advice; it is even better if this comes from people who have successfully completed this type of diet. But that doesn't mean that you shouldn't listen to friendly advice from other people. Any useful information is considered advice, use it or don't; it is entirely up to you.

Chapter 3- 30-day meal plan

This chapter is all about the meal plans I have drawn up. This is a 30-day keto diet plan and has been proven successful for weight loss.

There are so many recipes that can fall into this meal plan, so don't be shy to do some research on how to make them. You will see that pizza and other greasy-like foods are still listed on this meal plan. This is because you can still make them with different ingredients from what the original recipe uses.

Day	Breakfast	Lunch	Dinner
Monday	Bacon spinach casserole	Spicy beef salad	Prawns zucchini linguini
Tuesday	Egg salad	Green beans pork stir fry	Burger pancakes
Wednesday	Oopsie bread breakfast sandwich	Smoked chicken salad	Pork bombs with brie
Thursday	Bacon egg cups	Chicken bacon crustless quiche	Smoked haddock casserole
Friday	Ham cheese rolls	Taco mince with crispy cheese	Meatballs in creamy tomato sauce
Saturday	Mini egg muffins	Cauliflower chicken cheesy skillet	Meatloaf
Sunday	Smoked pancetta	Tuna salad	Stuffed chicken rolls

	crustless quiche		
Day	Breakfast	Lunch	Dinner
Monday	Chia pudding	Shrimp and cauliflower salad	Low carb burgers
Tuesday	Devilled eggs	Spaghetti squash	Low carb pizza
Wednesday	Classic bacon and eggs	Chicken and mashed cauliflower	Salmon with pesto sauce
Thursday	Cauliflower hash browns	Portabella burgers	Steak and garlic kale
Friday	Omelettes	Low carb spaghetti	Eggplant pizza
Saturday	Lox and cream cheese on flax crackers	Garlic shrimp and spinach salad	Low carb lasagna
Sunday	Pancakes low carb style	Steak and mushroom lettuce wraps	Mozzarella meatballs
Day	Breakfast	Lunch	Dinner
Monday	Waffles low carb style	Turkey lettuce wraps	Shakshuka
Tuesday	Smoked salmon with cream cheese, tomato, and onion	Roast beef salad	Pizza frittata

Wednesday	Green smoothie	Bacon chef's salad	Tuna casserole

Thursday	Egg with salsa and cheese	Low carb chilli with beef	Steak and potato salad
Friday	Egg bake and skillets with meat and veggies	Bacon crunch brussels sprouts	Zucchini shrimp scampi
Saturday	Peanut butter on flax crackers	Chicken and zucchini poppers	Low carb lettuce wrap tacos
Sunday	Guacamole and bacon with eggs	Low carb french fries	Low carb stuffed peppers
Day	Breakfast	Lunch	Dinner
Monday	Lox and cream cheese on flax crackers	Zucchini patties	Strawberry spinach chicken salad
Tuesday	Tuna salad on cucumbers	Baked salmon with lemon garlic butter	Pork roast with crispy asparagus
Wednesday	Coconut porridge	Bacon mushroom cheeseburger lettuce wraps	Chicken breast with herb butter
Thursday	Oopsie bread breakfast sandwich	Stuffed tomatoes	Mozzarella mushroom and chicken bake

Friday	Bacon egg cups	Low carb meat pie	Sushi feast
Saturday	Ham cheese rolls	Steak with bearnaise sauce	Lamb roast with herbs and cream cheese
Sunday	Mini egg muffins	Grilled polish sausage with	Low carb chicken
		cabbage	quesadillas

Remember, at the beginning of chapter one, I mentioned that you might not see much of a difference in the first two weeks. This is completely normal. Don't give up, because like I said, these things take time. Try your best and don't get discouraged.

These foods don't taste bad at all, and they are worth your time to prepare. You will begin to have a lot more energy and you will wake up in a better mood than you usually would. In order for you to mentally and physically accept this lifestyle, you need to think of this as a treat to your body.

It doesn't help if you feel like you are being punished. A negative mindset and pessimistic thoughts are not going to help you at all. You need to do your best to remain positive. Remember you are doing this for yourself.

Chapter 4- The science behind the keto weight loss

At the beginning of this book, I mentioned that we need energy to keep us alive. The reason we eat food is so that our bodies can break it down and turn it into useable energy, which will in turn keep us energized throughout the day.

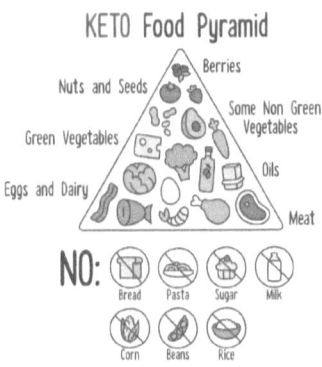

The human body is an amazing thing. A lot of its energy is stored in the body's fats and ketones. Your body also retrieves the glucose from the liver and all your carbohydrates from the food you eat.

Now you might recall what happens when we take away carbohydrates; that's right, your body will reach a state of ketosis.

After you eat any food containing carbohydrates, and it has entered your bloodstream, it is readily broken down into what we call glucose. Then, your body's insulin steps in to try and remove all the excess glucose from your bloodstream. It then takes your glucose and turns it into glycogen, which is stored primarily in your body's muscles.

All the stored glycogen then can cause problems if you don't exercise regularly. It runs out of space in the muscles and uses the last space in the liver, your liver will then send out a signal to stop the production of insulin.

It is at this point that the glycogen has nowhere to go, so more and more insulin is distributed into your bloodstream, and this without a doubt leads to insulin resistance. When your body is at this point, the liver transfers any left-over glucose to be stored as body fat.

This is when you start to gain weight and develop type 2 diabetes as well as many other metabolic issues.

This is the beauty of this diet; this diet reprograms your body and can even help with common illnesses such as polycystic ovarian syndrome and irritable bowel syndrome.

Typically ketones have no role in giving the body energy or producing it either. For those of you who don't know what ketones and ketone bodies are, I am going to provide you with a definition by Wikipedia, along with a simple interpretation as it can get a little confusing ("Ketone bodies," n.d.).

"Ketone bodies have three molecules (acetoacetate, beta-hydroxybutyrate and the spontaneous breakdown product of acetoacetate, acetone) containing the ketone group that is formed by the liver by fatty acids during periods of low food intake, restrictive carbohydrate diets, starvation, lengthy forceful exercise, boozing or in untreated type 1 diabetes."

To sum that up in simple terms, ketones are produced by the liver during a normal carbohydrate diet, which is similar to fasting for long periods of time.

"Ketone bodies are willingly transported into tissues outside the liver and converted into acetyl-CoA, which then enters the citric acid cycle and is oxidised in the mitochondria for energy. In the brain, ketone bodies are also used to make acetyl-CoA into long-chain fatty acids."

Ketone bodies are transported into tissues and then converted into a long chain of fatty acids.

"Ketone bodies are formed by the liver under the circumstances listed above as a product of powerful gluconeogenesis, which is the production of glucose from non-carbohydrate sources."

"They are thus continuously unrestricted into the blood by the liver together with newly formed glucose after the liver glycogen stores have been exhausted; this happens within the first 24 hours."

"When two acetyl-CoA molecules lose their A groups they can form a (covalent) dinner called acetoacetate. Beta-hydroxybutyrate remains a compact system of acetoacetate, in which the ketone group is transformed into an alcohol group."

"Both are four carbon molecules, that can eagerly be changed back into acetyl-CoA by utmost tissues of the body, with the distinguished allowance of the liver. Acetone is the

34

decarboxylated form of acetoacetate which cannot be converted back into acetyl-CoA except via detoxification in the liver where it is converted into lactic acid, which can, in turn, be oxidised into pyruvic acid, and only then into acetyl-CoA."

"Ketone bodies have a distinctive smell, which can easily be spotted in the smell of persons in ketosis and ketoacidosis. It is often labelled as fruity or like nail polish remover (which usually contains acetone or ethyl acetate)."

"Apart from the three endogenous ketone bodies, acetone, acetoacetic acid, and betahydroxybutyric acid, other ketone bodies like beta-keto pentanoate and betahydroxypentanoate possibly will be formed as a result of the metabolism of synthetic triglycerides, such as triheptanoin."

Ketone and ketone bodies are not the same thing. ketones, as defined by Wikipedia, are:

"In chemistry, a ketone is an animate compound with the structure RC(=O)R', where R and R' can be an assortment of carbon-containing substituents. Ketones and aldehydes are pure compounds that contain a carbonyl group (a carbon-oxygen double bond).

They are considered 'simple' because they do not have reactive groups like $-OH$ or $-Cl$ attached directly to the carbon atom in the carbonyl group, as in carboxylic acids containing $-COOH$. Many ketones are acknowledged, and many are of high position in the industry and in biology. Examples include many sugars (ketoses) and the manufacturing solvent acetone, which is the smallest ketone" ("Ketones," n.d.).

Lipolysis and Ketosis

Under normal circumstances, ketones have no business giving the body energy. But when you are on the keto diet, ketones are in charge of energy levels, and at the same time, start the automatic fat burning switch.

When carbs vanish, the body goes into a state called lipolysis, which is scientifically proven to be in direct correlation with weight loss. The body is forced to use the fat stored in your muscles and melts it off the body, which is referred to as ketosis.

Ketosis and keto acids are two different concepts. Ketosis is a natural fat burning process while keto acids is what arises in diabetes; that is why keto acids are very dangerous (Lis, 2019).

Benefits of the Ketogenic Diet

There is an overwhelming amount of advantages you can get from this diet and lifestyle. The first advantage is weight loss. It has been proven in a number of studies that eating low carbs results in weight loss. This has been verified by the thousands of people, like me, who have struggled with weight.

Keto diet eliminates cravings you have on a day to day basis. It stabilizes your blood sugar levels and your appetite. It also lowers your levels of visceral fat, which is your belly fat and the excess fat surrounding your organs. As a result, your blood pressure will also be lowered, which will make it less likely that you experience a stroke or heart attack.

Keto diet also has the benefit of reducing the risk of heart disease, diabetes, and cancer. This diet is also used to treat several types of cancer and slows down the growth of tumours in the body. It is also used to treat brain injury, Parkinson's disease, epilepsy, Alzheimer's disease, and Polycystic ovarian syndrome (Lis, 2019).

The ketogenic diet increases your protein intake, which has a lot of benefits for your body. It also limits your carbohydrate consumption, which means you have a smaller variety of foods to choose from to eat, resulting in weight loss.

Chapter 5 - Increasing your metabolism on the keto diet

When you start the keto diet, you might feel like your metabolism has taken a step back. There is nothing to worry about because this section is here for if you need it. There are also strips you can buy to test your level of ketosis, which will help you determine what your metabolism is like at its current stage.

Once you see that you are in the ketosis phase, this means that your metabolism is at its best it can be. If the results are opposite of that, that is when you look for ways to kick start your metabolism in order to reach ketosis. Below are seven tips you can follow to try and reach your desired level of ketosis (Fletcher, 2019).

Let's take a look at these and remember, if you keep eating correctly, there will not be a need to do this. If you are struggling, then I am here to help you.

1. Increase your physical activity

This one is first on the list because it's most important. In the beginning, I told you to take it easy unless you get the go-ahead from your doctor or personal trainer. If you haven't reached somewhere close to ketosis within the first month and a half, there is a possibility that you are not exercising enough.

2. Reducing carbohydrate intake

If you decided to start the diet off with just 20 grams of carbs a day, you might want to cut that down to about half. It is possible that your body is still consuming too many carbohydrates and that will, without a doubt, cause a problem with your metabolism. So, reduce your carb intake.

3. Fasting for short periods

If you haven't decided to fast yet, now might be a good time to do this. Start off fasting one day a week and see what that does for you. If you see no changes, increase it two days a week but don't fast one day after the other; this can be dangerous. Fast for short periods of time. I'm sure that if you do this, you will be able to see the results.

4. Increase your healthy fats

It's important you include foods in your diet that are considered healthy fats. An example of healthy fats are an avocado and nuts. You can also cook food using flaxseed oil, coconut oil, or a basic virgin olive oil.

5. Test your ketone levels

You can have your ketones tested through a blood test. A blood test may not be your only option, but it is by far the easiest. A blood test will give you all the information you need. Get a blood test form from your general practitioner and visit your nearest blood clinic; it's that easy!

6. Maintain a high protein intake

Remember what I mentioned earlier about watching your protein intake and levels. If you are still struggling with this, it's likely that you are not getting enough protein to sustain ketosis. You will lose muscle mass instead of gaining, and that should be your first warning sign.

7. Use coconut oil

This is an excellent investment. The easiest way to reach ketosis is through the use of coconut oil. This one goes hand in hand with tip #4. If you do both correctly, you won't have a problem reaching your weight goals. Coconut oil isn't very hard to find, and it's generally inexpensive. It's very good for you, and it will make your life a hell of a lot easier.

Generally, if you have reached ketosis, you already know that you simply have to follow the same routine every day. However, we are all human and we sometimes make mistakes, and that's totally okay.

Remaining positive throughout your journey

There will be days where you will feel like none of this is worth it and that you are wasting your time. However, I can promise you that it will all be worth it in the end.

Male or female, come hell or high water I have faith in you, and I believe you can do this! If you are really struggling with motivation, set yourself a goal board. Take an A5 piece of cardboard and stick your goals on there, so that every time you feel like giving up, you will be reminded of what you are working towards.

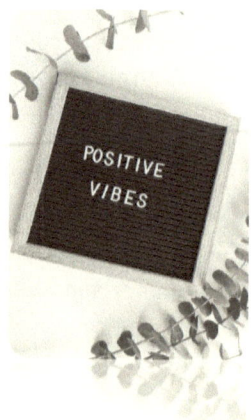

I can proudly say I lost over 20 kilograms after adopting this lifestyle, and I have never felt better. I don't feel like I lack energy, and I am actually excited to wake up in the mornings because I feel good about myself.

This lifestyle has wholly built up my self-image, and I have finally escaped the depression that had been weighing me down for 19 years. Your mental health is just as important as your physical health, so it's important you take charge of your life now.

Many people these days suffer from low self-esteem, and I can guarantee that at one point in your life, you have felt terrible about yourself. But once you start losing all that extra weight, you start to feel really good about yourself.

Clothes that used to be too small will now fit comfortably, and you will be able to live a long and healthy life the same way that I am. It makes the world's difference, so go and grab some paper and cut out pictures for inspiration and motivation or write down your goals.

Every time you want to give up and throw in the towel, just know that this is a normal reaction, but once you get past that, you will see that the results will change your life forever.

10 things you need to know about the keto diet

As with any diet, there are things you need to know beforehand. Things that you might find strange but that are completely normal. The following list will provide you with 10 additional facts about the keto diet ("The Top 10 Things," 2019):

1. Keto can treat medical conditions

As you might recall, a keto diet can in fact treat grave medical conditions.

2. Eating keto foods doesn't have to be expensive

Some diets can become very expensive; however, a keto diet doesn't have to be. Now that you have a list of what you can and can not eat, you can go and buy your ingredients in bulk, thereby saving money.

3. Keto is more than just a diet

This is true on so many levels. It helps manage diseases such as those listed earlier in the book. It's not just a diet, and it's also not something you can start then stop; it becomes a part of your lifestyle.

4. Keto customization

You can adjust your keto diet to the way your body works and how your body processes carbohydrates. You need to figure out what works for you and stick to it.

5. Keto takes time

As I have mentioned so many times already, it might take a few days before you notice any changes. All the stories you hear of people dropping weight like it's hot is simply because they had more excess weight to lose than you do. So, be patient.

6. Ketosis is different for everyone

Unfortunately, no human being's body works in the same way; so no two people will lose the same amount of weight at the same time. This is physically impossible.

7. Keto flu is a real thing

You think you might be picking up the flu, right? Wrong! This is your body's way of adjusting to the change. You might feel sore and feel like you have the flu, but you really do not.

8. Keto breath is real

The scent of your breath will change as it adapts to your new lifestyle. Some have described the smell to be similar to acetone (nail polish remover). Remember to brush those pearly whites and carry around breath mints; it's a small price to pay!

9. Keto will affect your workouts

Like I said previously, in the beginning stages of the diet, complete your workouts at a low intensity. If you were a daily exerciser prior to the keto diet,, the speed at which you complete exercises will change and you may become slower. However, it will get a lot easier as you progress further into your diet. So, don't worry, you'll get to the intensity you were once at really soon.

10. Keto farts

This diet can cause a build-up of a lot of gas. Depending on who you are and what you eat, the intensity will vary. Your stomach will be adjusting, so don't be surprised by the gas.

Conclusion

Now that we have reached the end of our journey together, I would like to take this opportunity to thank you for taking the time for me to give you all the valuable information that you need on your keto journey.

Let's review everything that we have covered, right from the very start.

- Keto diet and weight loss tips

1. Be persistent
2. Avoid fruit
3. Eat only when hungry
4. Review your medicine
5. Eat less dairy and nuts
6. Supplement vitamins and minerals
7. Support during your journey
8. Exercise
9. Check your hormones
10. Avoid your weekend beer
11. Choose a low carb diet
12. Determine if you are really hungry
13. Stress less
14. Sleep correctly
15. Intermittent fasting
16. Track your progress

As you can see, we have come a very long way together. If this process is followed, the success rate is 100%. All you need is motivation and a love for the lifestyle.

With all of this information, you are guaranteed to lose weight and become another success story. Remember to be patient with yourself.

If you are one of the lucky ones, you will lose most of your excess weight within the first week. Remember to take it easy with your exercises and don't be afraid to eat your food.

Remember to check in with a professional to make sure that this diet is suitable for you depending on your current health.

The keto lifestyle isn't for everyone. But if you push through, you will receive all the benefits and more.

Don't give up on yourself, remember your goal board, and don't get discouraged when results don't appear as quickly as you'd like them to.

Remember that once your 30 days are up, you can go and look for other keto-friendly recipes so you can enjoy your food, your life, and the brand new you!

Citations

Ayuda, T. (2019). 10 Calorie-Torching Exercises to Do If You Want to Lose Weight. [online] Prevention. Available at: https://www.prevention.com/weight-loss/a20474562/bestweight-loss-exercises/ [Accessed 20 May 2019].

Dr. Andreas Eenfeldt, M. (2019). How to Lose Weight – The Top 18 Simple Tips – Diet Doctor. [online] Diet Doctor. Available at: https://www.dietdoctor.com/how-to-lose-weight#2 [Accessed 20 May 2019].

Dr. Anthony Gustin, M. (2019). 47 Healthy Keto Snacks That Won't Kick You Out of Ketosis. [online] Perfect Keto. Available at: https://perfectketo.com/ultimate-healthy-keto-snacklist/ [Accessed 20 May 2019].

Pixabay.com. (2019). Free Image on Pixabay - Acetone, Ketone, Carbonyl Group. [online] Available at: https://pixabay.com/illustrations/acetone-ketone-carbonyl-group-2876278/ [Accessed 20 May 2019].

Pixabay.com. (2019). Free Image on Pixabay - Food, Diet, Keto, Ketodieta. [online] Available at: https://pixabay.com/photos/food-diet-keto-ketodieta-fitness-3223286/ [Accessed 20 May 2019].

Pixabay.com. (2019). Free Image on Pixabay - Salad, Fresh, Food, Diet, Health. [online] Available at: https://pixabay.com/photos/salad-fresh-food-diet-health-374173/ [Accessed 20 May 2019].

Pixabay.com. (2019). Free Image on Pixabay - Smiley, Emoticon, Dash Face, Grin. [online] Available at: https://pixabay.com/illustrations/smiley-emoticon-dash-face-grin-1020193/ [Accessed 20 May 2019].

Pixabay.com. (2019). Free Image on Pixabay - Yoga, Meditation, Spiritual, Mental. [online] Available at: https://pixabay.com/vectors/yoga-meditation-spiritual-mental-153436/ [Accessed 20 May 2019].

Frey, M. (2019). The 3 Types of Exercise You Need to Lose Weight. [online] Verywell Fit. Available at: https://www.verywellfit.com/types-of-exercise-for-weight-loss-3495992 [Accessed 20 May 2019].

Katherine Marengo LDN, R. (2019). 7 fast and effective ways to get into ketosis. [online] Medical News Today. Available at: https://www.medicalnewstoday.com/articles/324599.php [Accessed 20 May 2019].

En.wikipedia.org. (2019). Ketone. [online] Available at: https://en.wikipedia.org/wiki/Ketone [Accessed 20 May 2019].

En.wikipedia.org. (2019). Ketone bodies. [online] Available at: https://en.wikipedia.org/wiki/Ketone_bodies [Accessed 20 May 2019].

Lis, N. (2019, January 03). Keto Diet Guide for Beginners. Retrieved from https://lowcarbbabe.com/keto-diet-guide-beginners-download/

Morgan, H. (2019). Importance of Living a Healthy Lifestyle | Livestrong.com. [online] LIVESTRONG.COM. Available at: https://www.livestrong.com/article/31783-importancelifestyle/ [Accessed 20 May 2019].

Scott, J. (2019). Getting a Workout in the Pool Can Be Easy for Beginners. [online] Verywell Fit. Available at: https://www.verywellfit.com/swimming-for-beginners-weight-lossadvice-3496001 [Accessed 20 May 2019].

KetoLogic. (2019). The Top 10 Things You Need to Know Before Going Keto - KetoLogic. [online] Available at: https://ketologic.com/article/the-top-10-things-you-need-to-knowbefore-going-keto/ [Accessed 20 May 2019].

If you like go to Amazon and leave a review of the book!

Thank you and good luck!

www.ingramcontent.com/pod-product-compliance
Lightning Source LLC
Chambersburg PA
CBHW020331290526
45785CB00007B/3011